The Daniel Fast Diet

Including 25 Delicious 15-Minute Recipes for Fasting

Disclaimer and Terms of Use:

Effort has been made to ensure that the information in this book is accurate and complete, however, the author and the publisher do not warrant the accuracy of the information, text and graphics contained within the book due to the rapidly changing nature of science, research, known and unknown facts and internet. The Author and the publisher do not hold any responsibility for errors, omissions or contrary interpretation of the subject matter herein. This book is presented solely for motivational and informational purposes only.

Table of Contents

Introduction

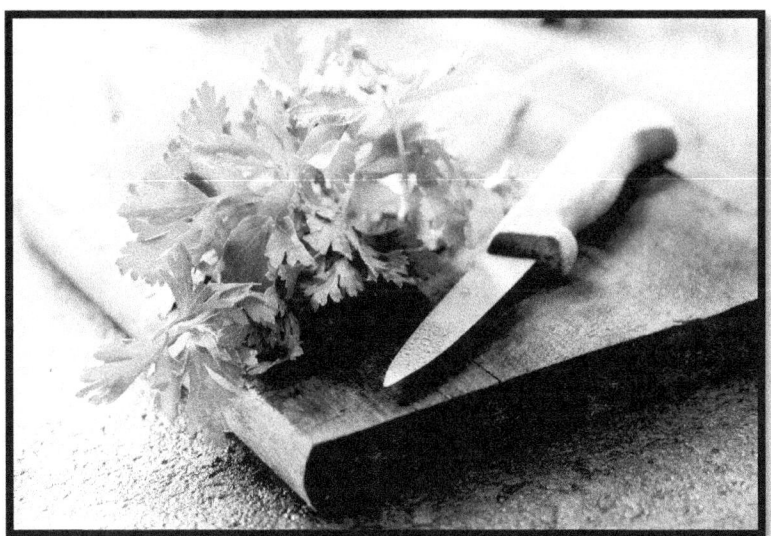

By now you are probably familiar with dozens of types of diets. Many of them are created by celebrities to promote their brand or even by health professionals to combat certain health problems. The Daniel Fast Diet is in a category all its own because its roots come from the Bible itself. In the book of Daniel, the prophet named Daniel chooses to honor God by engaging in a fast during which he restricts himself to consuming only fruits, vegetables, and water. At the end of his fast, Daniel and his companions are found to be in good health – stronger, in fact, than the king of Babylon's warriors who consumed rich foods and wine. If you are looking for a way to improve your nutrition and, as an optional spiritual element to the diet, strengthen your relationship with God, the Daniel Fast Diet is a great choice.

When starting a new diet, it can take time to get used to the rules and restrictions you have to follow. On top of this challenge is the difficulty of finding the time to prepare a healthy meal for your whole family to enjoy. That is where this book comes in. In addition to providing you with an introduction to the Daniel Fast Diet, you will also receive a collection of quick and easy Daniel Fast Diet recipes that the whole family will love. From tasty breakfasts like Sautéed Sweet Potato Hash to filling dinners like Homemade Tomato Basil Pasta, the recipes in this book will introduce you to the Daniel Fast Diet and get you hooked. So what are you waiting for? Pick a recipe and start cooking today!

Delicious Daniel Fast Diet Recipes

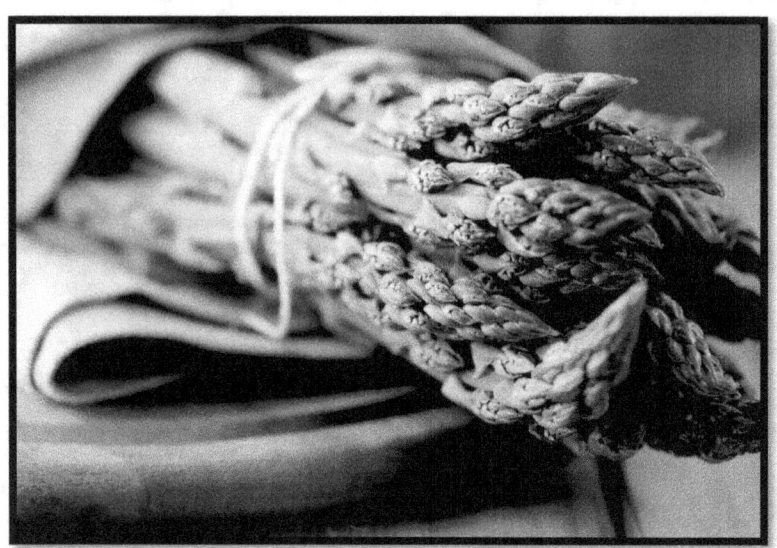

Recipes Included in this Book:

Servings: 4

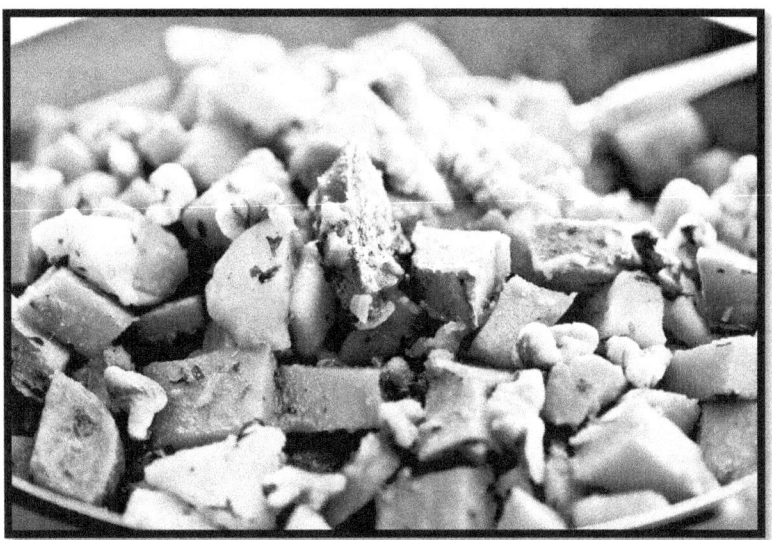

Ingredients:

2 tablespoons coconut oil

2 large sweet potatoes, peeled and chopped

½ medium onion, chopped

1 cup chopped cauliflower florets

¼ cup chopped walnut halves

1 teaspoon minced garlic

1 teaspoon chili powder

Salt and pepper to taste

Instructions:

1. Heat the oil in a large skillet over medium-high heat.
2. Add the sweet potato and stir to coat with oil then add 2 tablespoons water and cover the skillet.
3. Steam the sweet potato for 3 to 4 minutes then stir in the onion, garlic and cauliflower.
4. Cook for 5 to 7 minutes, stirring often, until the onion is translucent and the sweet potato tender.
5. Stir in the walnuts, chili powder, salt and pepper then serve hot.

Servings: 1 to 2

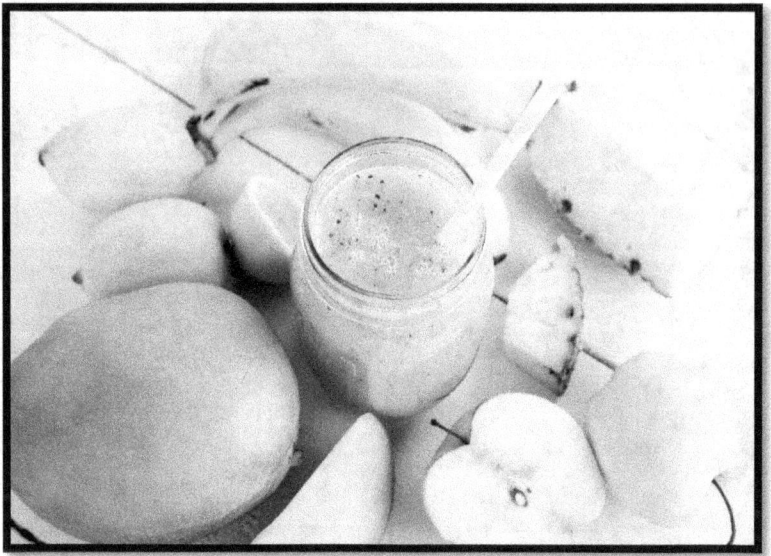

Ingredients:

1 cup frozen chopped mango

1 cup frozen chopped pineapple

1 small frozen banana, peeled and sliced

1 cup organic orange juice

½ cup ice cubes

¼ cup canned coconut milk

1 tablespoon fresh lemon juice

Instructions:

1. Combine all of the ingredients in a high-speed blender.
2. Blend on high speed for 30 to 60 seconds until smooth and well combined.
3. Pour into a large glass and enjoy immediately.

Servings: 6

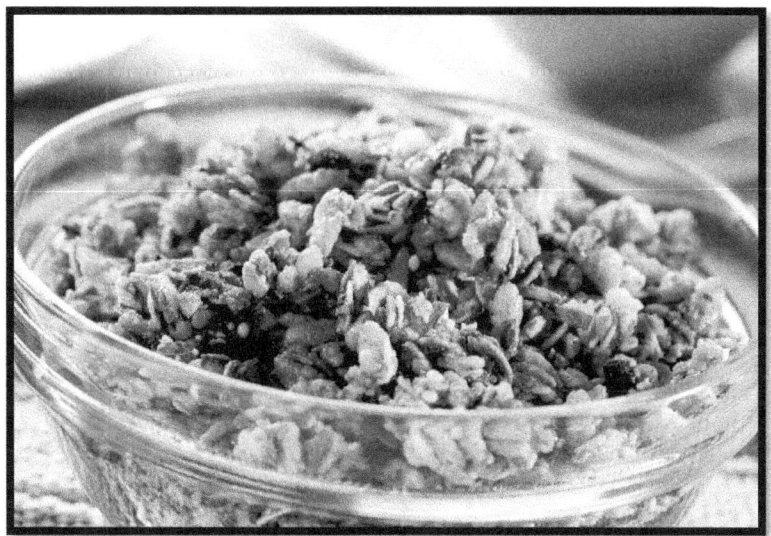

Ingredients:

3 cups old-fashioned oats
2 cups unsweetened coconut flakes
½ cup pecans
½ cup chopped walnuts
1/3 cup coconut oil, melted
1 teaspoon vanilla extract
½ teaspoon ground cinnamon
Pinch salt
1 to 1 ½ cups seedless raisins

Instructions:

1. Preheat the oven to 325°F.
2. Combine the oats, coconut flakes, pecans, and walnuts in a mixing bowl.
3. In a separate bowl, whisk together the coconut oil, vanilla extract, cinnamon and salt.
4. Drizzle the oil mixture over the oat mixture and toss well to coat then spread evenly on a large baking sheet.
5. Bake for 12 to 15 minutes until golden brown, stirring once in a while.
6. Transfer the toasted oat mixture to a large bowl and stir in the raisins to serve.

Servings: 1

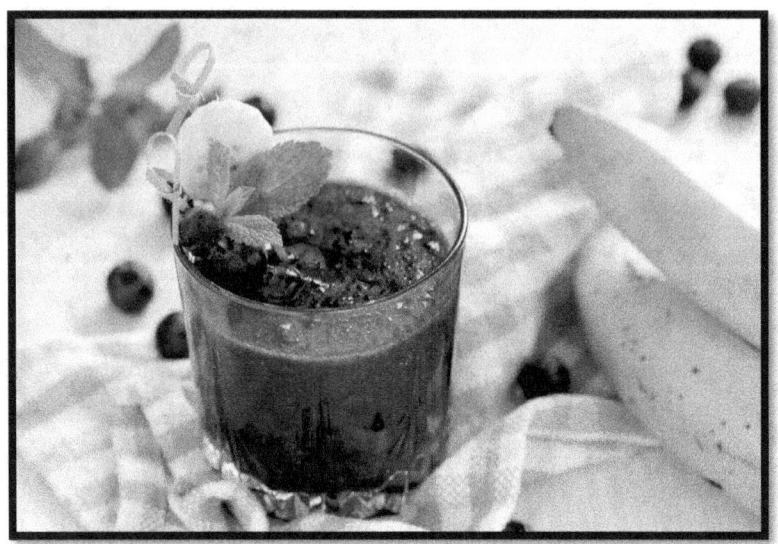

Ingredients:

1 ½ cups frozen blueberries
1 large frozen banana, peeled and sliced
1 cup unsweetened almond milk
½ cup ice cubes
¼ cup canned coconut milk

Instructions:

1. Combine all of the ingredients in a high-speed blender.
2. Blend on high speed for 30 to 60 seconds until smooth and well combined.
3. Pour into a large glass and enjoy immediately.

Servings: 4

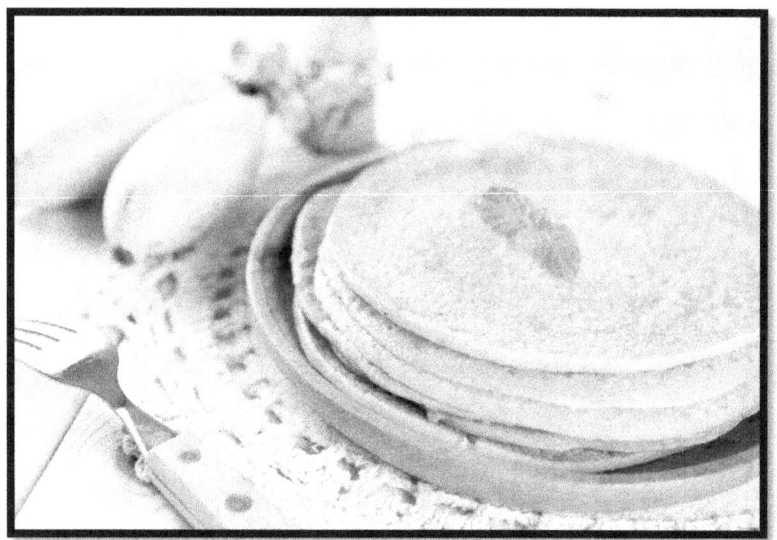

Ingredients:

2 tablespoons ground flaxseed

2/3 cup warm water

5 tablespoons coconut flour

1 ¼ teaspoons baking powder

Pinch salt

1 cup unsweetened almond milk

1 teaspoon vanilla extract

2 large bananas, peeled and mashed

Instructions:

1. Combine the ground flaxseed and warm water in a small bowl and whisk well then set aside for 5 minutes.
2. Meanwhile, combine the coconut flour, baking powder and salt in a mixing bowl.
3. In another bowl, whisk together the almond milk and vanilla extract then stir in the mashed bananas
4. Add the flax mixture and stir until well combined then add the dry ingredients in small batches, stirring until just combined.
5. Heat a large skillet over medium heat and grease with cooking spray.
6. Drop the batter onto the skillet using 2 to 3 tablespoons per pancake.

7. Cook the pancakes for 1 to 2 minutes until browned on the underside then flip and cook for another 1 to 2 minutes.
8. Transfer the pancakes to a plate to keep warm and repeat with the remaining batter.

Servings: 4

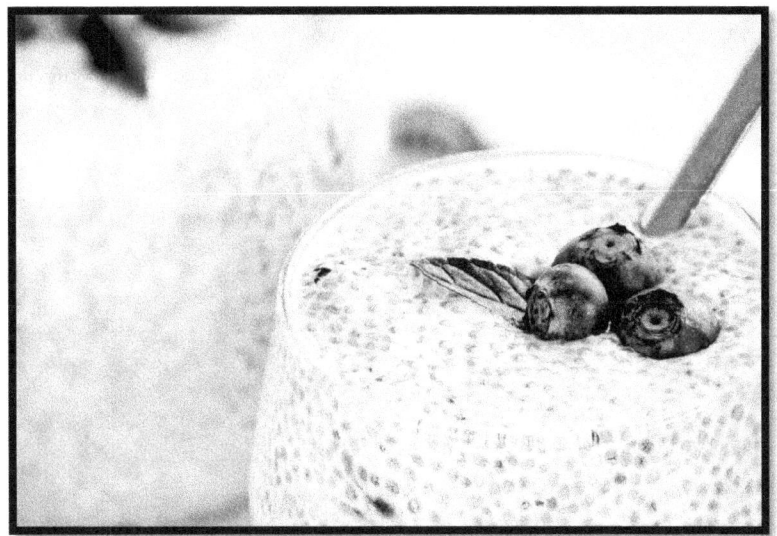

Ingredients:

1 ½ cups unsweetened coconut milk beverage

¼ cup chia seeds

1 teaspoon vanilla extract

Pinch salt

½ cup fresh blueberries

Instructions:

1. Combine the coconut milk with the chia seeds, vanilla extract and salt in a small mixing bowl.
2. Whisk together then cover and chill for 3 hours or so.
3. Spoon the pudding into small dessert cups and top with fresh blueberries.

Servings: 4

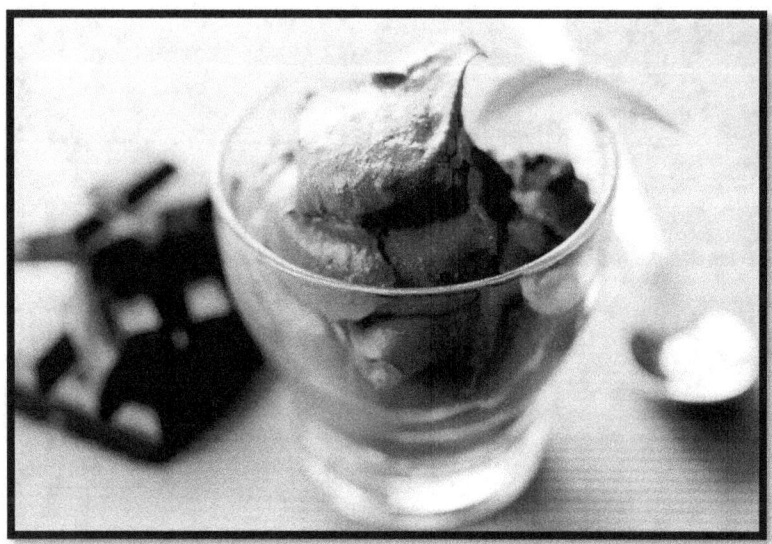

Ingredients:

2 large ripe avocadoes, pitted and chopped

1/3 cup unsweetened cocoa powder

2 tablespoons unsweetened almond milk

1 tablespoon chia seeds

1 teaspoon vanilla extract

Instructions:

1. Puree the avocado in a food processor then add the almond milk, cocoa powder, chia seeds, and vanilla extract.
2. Blend the mixture until smooth and well combined.
3. Spoon the mousse into small dessert cups and chill for 30 to 60 minutes before serving.

Coconut Date Balls

Servings: 24

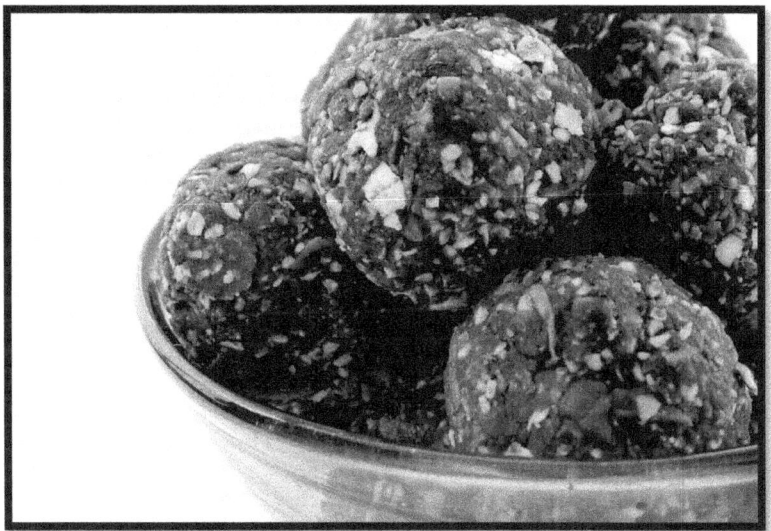

Ingredients:

2 cups raw cashews
1 cup unsweetened shredded coconut
2 tablespoons coconut oil
2 cups pitted Medjool dates
1 ¼ teaspoon vanilla extract
½ teaspoon salt

Instructions:

1. Combine the cashews and coconut in a food processor and blend until crumbled.
2. Add the coconut oil, dates, vanilla extract and salt.
3. Blend the mixture until it forms a sticky batter.
4. Scoop the batter out using a tablespoon and roll the batter into balls by hand.
5. Arrange the balls on a parchment-lined baking sheet and chill for at least 1 hour until firm.

Servings: 4

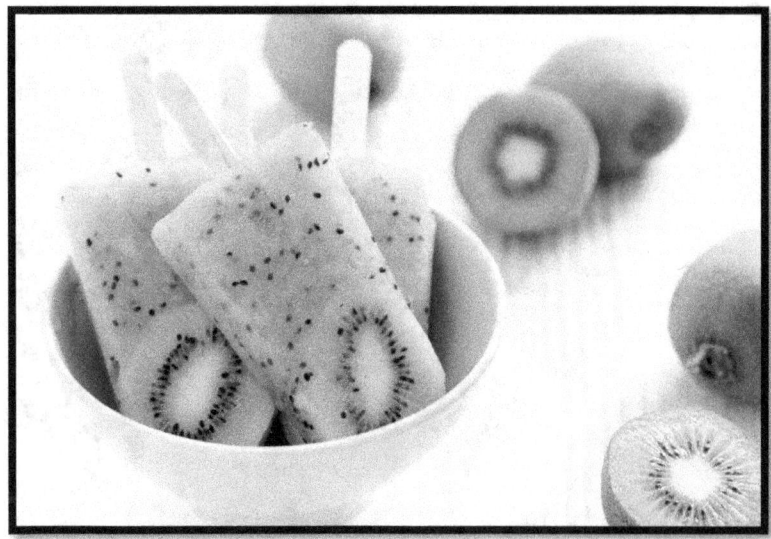

Ingredients:

5 ripe kiwifruit, peeled and sliced
1 ½ cups unsweetened pineapple juice

Instructions:

1. Reserve 4 slices of kiwi then place the rest in a food processor and blend until smooth.
2. Add the pineapple juice and blend again until smooth and well combined.
3. Drop one slice of kiwi into each popsicle mold then fill with the kiwi-pineapple mixture.
4. Freeze the popsicles until solid then enjoy.

Servings: yields 1 ½ cups

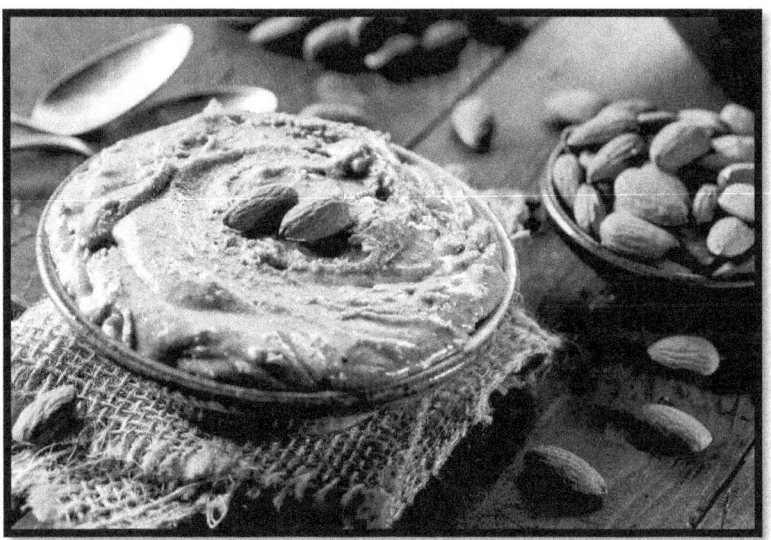

Ingredients:

3 cups raw almonds
Salt, if desired

Instructions:

1. Place the almonds in a food processor and secure the lid.
2. Blend the almonds for 15 minutes or so until smooth and creamy.
3. Season with salt, if desired.

Servings: 6 to 8

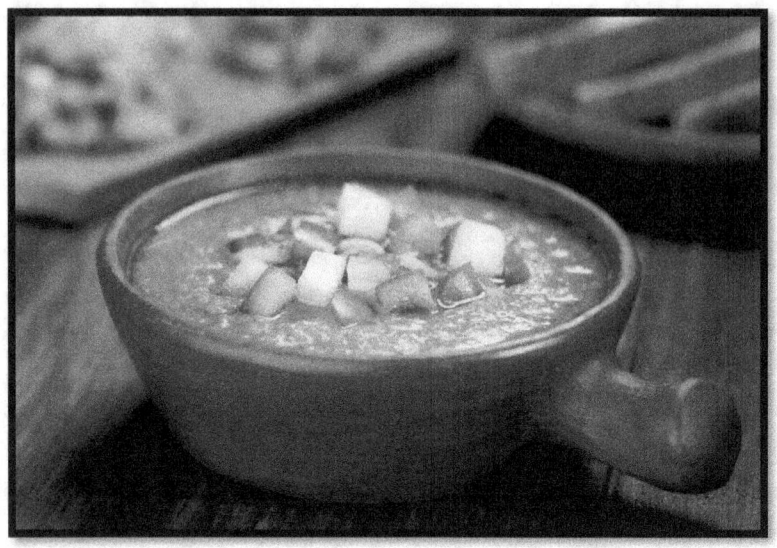

Ingredients:

3 cups coarsely chopped tomatoes
1 large seedless cucumber, chopped
1 large red bell pepper, cored and chopped
1 small red onion, chopped
3 cups organic tomato juice
¼ cup red wine vinegar
1 tablespoon minced garlic
2 tablespoons fresh lemon juice
1 tablespoon fresh chopped parsley
1 tablespoon fresh chopped cilantro
1 teaspoon fresh chopped thyme
Salt and pepper to taste

Instructions:

1. Place the tomato, cucumber, red pepper and red onion in a food processor.
2. Pulse the mixture until finely chopped but not pureed.
3. Remove ½ cup of the vegetable mixture and set aside then blend the rest until smooth.
4. Pour the vegetable puree into a mixing bowl and stir in the tomato juice, vinegar, garlic, lemon juice, and herbs.

5. Season with salt and pepper to taste then cover and chill for several hours.
6. Spoon the gazpacho into bowls and garnish with a tablespoon or so of the reserved chopped vegetables.

Servings:

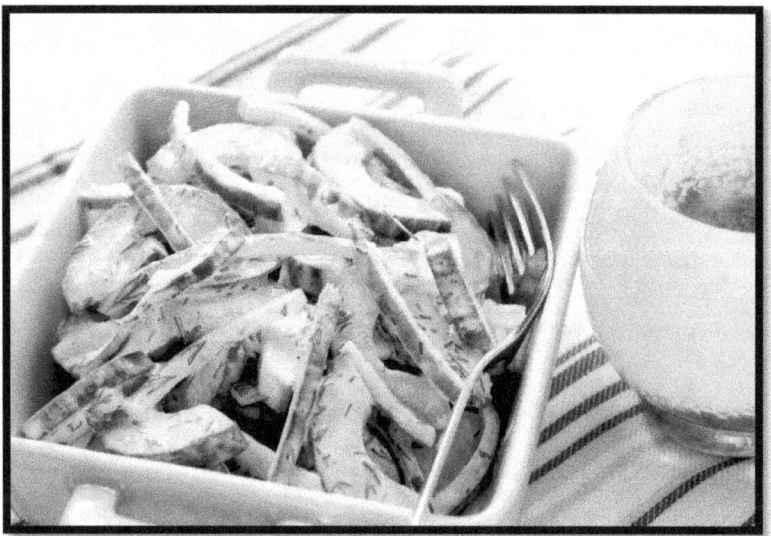

Ingredients:

¼ cup white-wine vinegar

2 tablespoons canned coconut milk

¼ teaspoon salt

2 tablespoons fresh chopped dill

2 large seedless cucumbers, sliced thin

½ medium red onion, sliced thin

Instructions:

1. Combine the vinegar, coconut milk, salt and dill in the bottom of a mixing bowl and stir well.
2. Add the cucumber and red onion, tossing to coat.
3. Cover and chill for several hours before serving.

Servings: 4

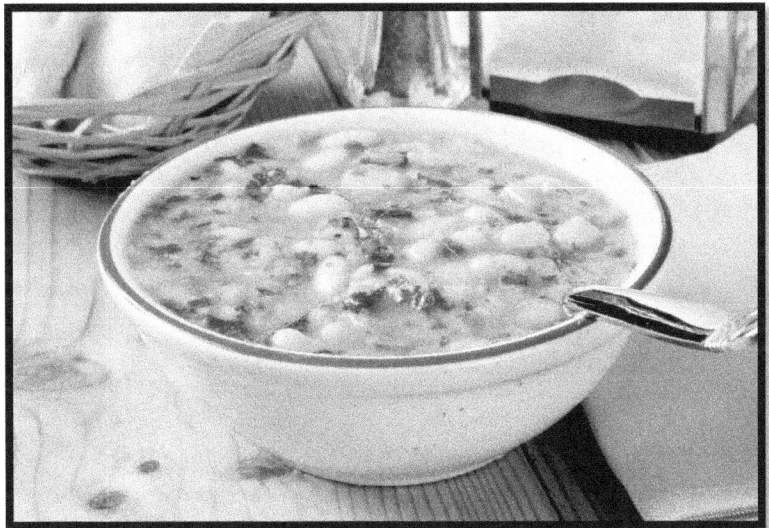

Ingredients:

1 tablespoon olive oil

1 cup diced yellow onion

1 tablespoon minced garlic

3 cups vegetable broth

2 (15.5 ounce) cans white cannellini beans, rinsed and drained

4 cups fresh chopped kale

Salt and pepper to taste

Instructions:

1. Heat the oil in a large saucepan over medium heat.
2. Add the onion and garlic then cook for 4 to 5 minutes until the onion is tender.
3. Stir in the vegetable broth and beans then bring to a boil.
4. Use a potato masher to partially mash the beans then stir in the kale.
5. Season with salt and pepper to taste and cook until heated through – about 5 minutes.

Servings: 4

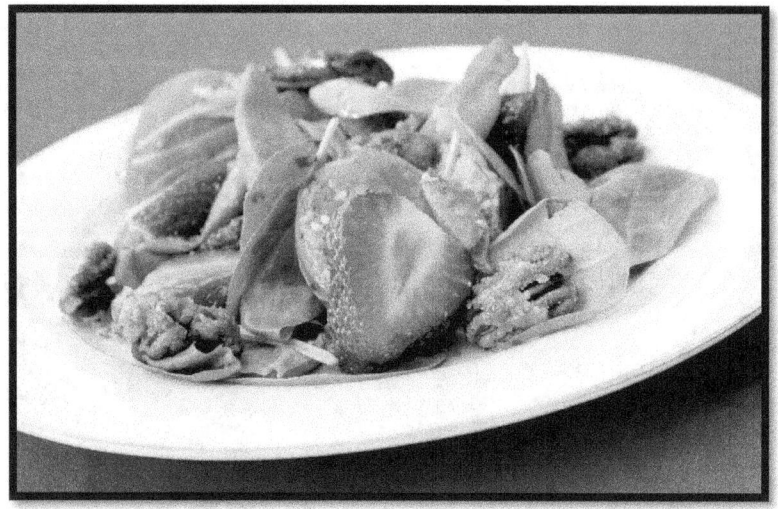

Ingredients:

6 cups fresh baby spinach
1 ½ cups fresh sliced strawberries
½ cup chopped walnut halves
¼ cup extra-virgin olive oil
2 tablespoons balsamic vinegar
1 teaspoon raspberry vinegar
Pinch dry mustard powder
Salt and pepper to taste

Instructions:

1. Divide the spinach among four salad plates and top each with strawberries and walnut halves.
2. Whisk together the remaining ingredients in a small bowl.
3. Drizzle the dressing over the salads to serve.

Servings: 4

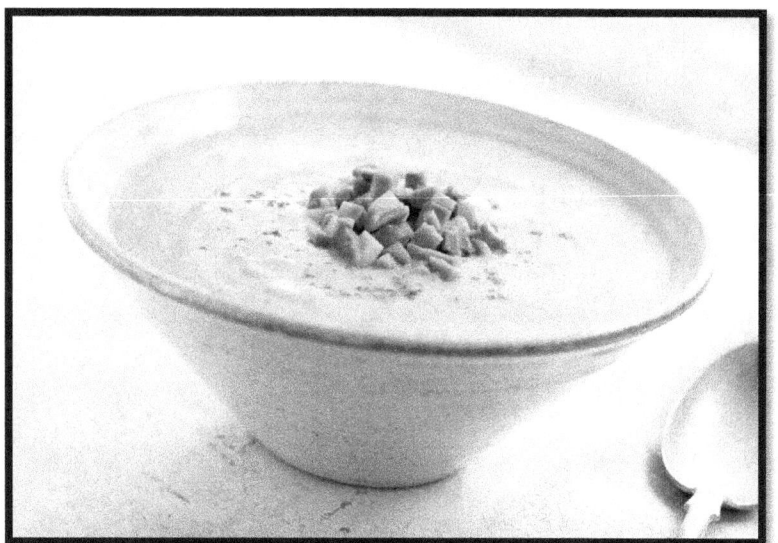

Ingredients:

2 large ripe avocado, pitted and chopped
2 cups vegetable broth
1 cup water
1 cup canned navy beans, rinsed and drained
½ cup canned coconut milk
2 tablespoons fresh lemon juice
Salt and pepper to taste
1 small jalapeno, seeded and minced

Instructions:

1. Combine the avocado, vegetable broth, water, navy beans and coconut milk in a food processor.
2. Blend until smooth and well combined then scrape down the sides of the bowl.
3. Add the lemon juice, salt, pepper and jalapeno and blend smooth.
4. Pour the soup into a bowl then cover and chill for 2 hours before serving.
5. Ladle the soup into bowls and serve garnished with diced avocado and a pinch of cayenne or paprika.

Servings: 6 to 8

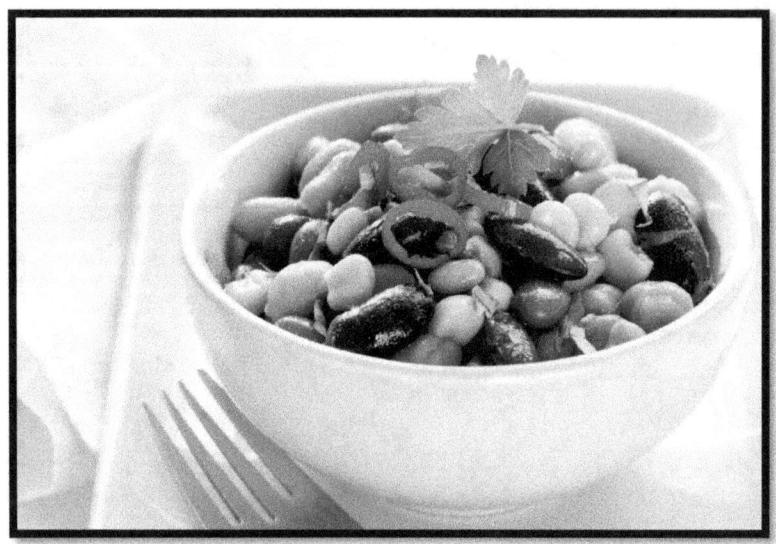

Ingredients:

1 (15 ounce) can red kidney beans, rinsed and drained

1 (15 ounce) can red white cannellini, rinsed and drained

1 (15 ounce) can red garbanzo beans, rinsed and drained

1 cup frozen corn, thawed

¼ cup diced red onion

2 stalks celery, diced very fine

¾ cup fresh chopped parsley

2 tablespoons fresh chopped dill

1/3 cup apple cider vinegar

¼ cup extra-virgin olive oil

2 tablespoons fresh lemon juice

Salt and pepper to taste

Instructions:

1. Combine the beans, corn, celery and onion in a mixing bowl.
2. Toss in the parsley and dill until well combined.
3. In a separate bowl, whisk together the remaining ingredients.
4. Drizzle the dressing over the salad and toss well to coat then chill until ready to serve – at least 2 hours.

Servings: 4

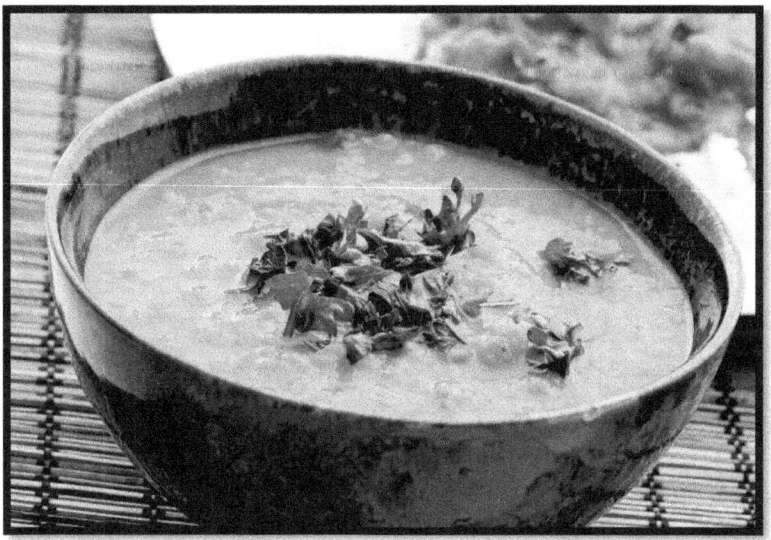

Ingredients:

1 tablespoon olive oil

1 cup diced yellow onion

1 tablespoon fresh grated ginger

3 cloves minced garlic

1 ½ tablespoons curry powder

3 cups vegetable broth

1 tablespoon balsamic vinegar

1lbs. steamed lentils

2 cups fresh chopped spinach

Salt and pepper to taste

Instructions:

1. Heat the oil in a large saucepan over medium heat.
2. Add the onion, garlic and ginger and cook for 4 to 5 minutes, stirring often.
3. Stir in the curry powder and cook for 30 seconds before whisking in the vegetable broth, vinegar and lentils.
4. Bring the soup to boil then reduce heat and simmer for 5 minutes.
5. Transfer half of the soup to a food processor and blend smooth.
6. Stir the blended lentils back into the saucepan along with the spinach then season with salt and pepper to taste.

Servings: 4

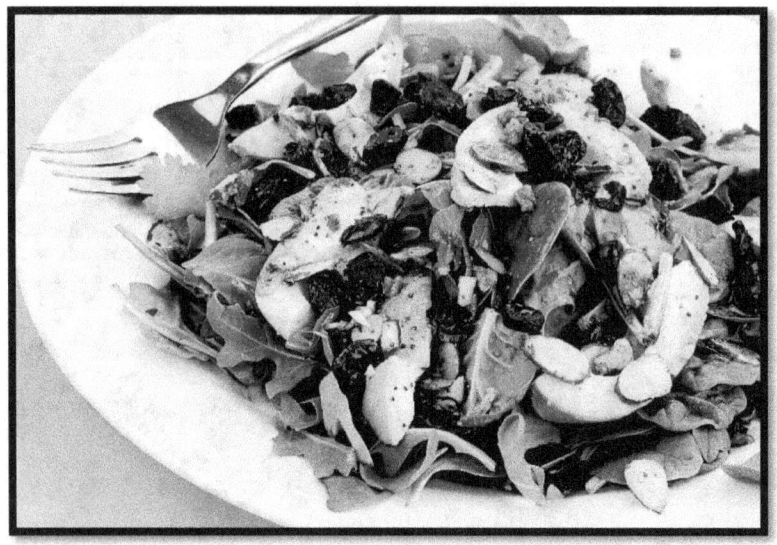

Ingredients:

6 cups fresh spring greens
1 large ripe avocado, pitted and sliced thin
½ cup seedless raisins
¼ cup thinly sliced almonds
¼ cup extra-virgin olive oil
2 tablespoons balsamic vinegar
1 teaspoon red wine vinegar
1 tablespoon minced white onion
½ clove garlic, minced
Salt and pepper to taste

Instructions:

1. Divide the greens among four salad plates and top each with slices of fresh avocado.
2. Sprinkle the salads with raisins and sliced almonds.
3. Add the remaining ingredients to a food processor and blend until smooth.
4. Drizzle the dressing over the salads to serve.

Servings: 4

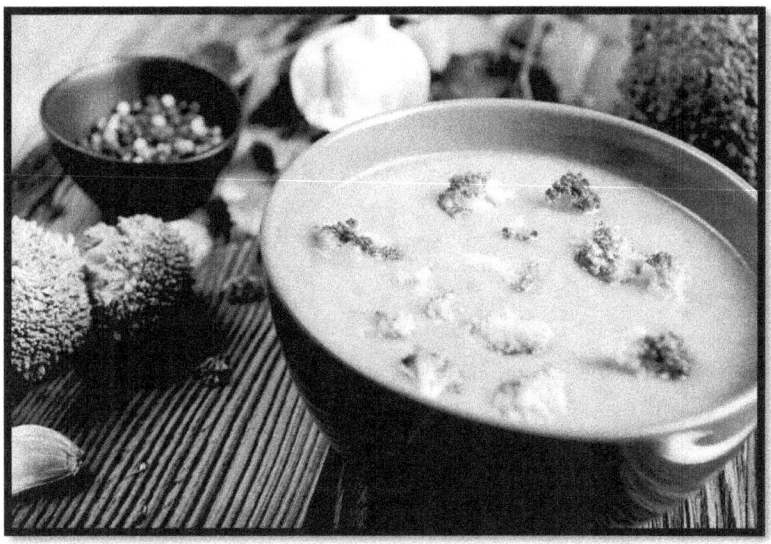

Ingredients:

8 cups fresh chopped broccoli florets
2 cups vegetable broth
1 cup canned coconut milk
Salt and pepper to taste

Instructions:

1. Bring a large pot of salted water to boil and add the broccoli.
2. Cook the broccoli for about 5 minutes until tender and bright green in color.
3. Drain the broccoli and set aside.
4. Combine the broth and coconut milk in a large saucepan and bring the mixture to a boil.
5. Stir in the broccoli then puree the soup using an immersion blender until smooth and well combined.
6. Season with salt and pepper to taste.

Servings: 4

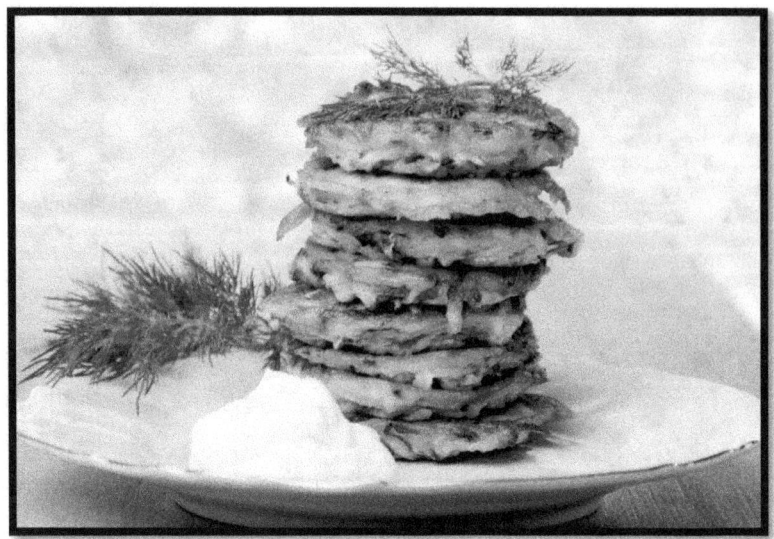

Ingredients:

1 large zucchini, grated
Salt, as needed
¼ cup ground almond meal
1 tablespoon coconut oil
2 cloves minced garlic
Salt and pepper to taste
Olive oil, as needed

Instructions:

1. Place the zucchini in a colander and sprinkle liberally with salt.
2. Let rest for 10 minutes then spread the zucchini on a clean towel and wring out as much moisture as possible.
3. Transfer the zucchini to a mixing bowl and stir in the almond meal, garlic, coconut oil, salt and pepper.
4. Heat a large skillet over medium heat and grease with olive oil.
5. Scoop the batter into the skillet using 2 to 3 tablespoons per fritter and fry for 2 minutes on each side until golden brown.
6. Drain on paper towels and repeat with the remaining batter.

Servings: 4

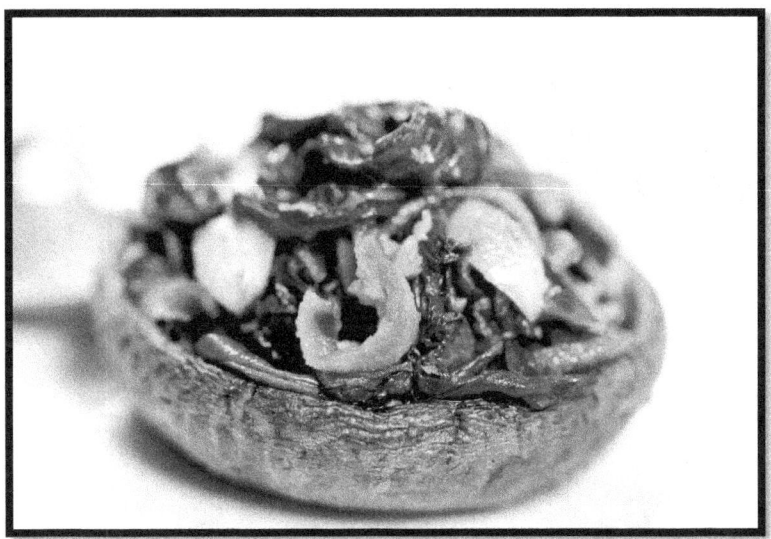

Ingredients:

4 large Portobello mushroom caps, stems removed
Olive oil, as need
3 cloves garlic, minced
1 small yellow onion, chopped
1 (10 ounce) package frozen spinach, thawed
Salt and pepper to taste

Instructions:

1. Preheat the broiler to high and line a baking sheet with foil.
2. Brush the mushroom caps with oil on both sides then broil for 3 to 4 minutes on each side until tender.
3. Heat 2 teaspoons oil in a large skillet over medium heat and add the garlic and onion.
4. Place the thawed spinach in a colander and press out as much moisture as possible.
5. Cook for 4 to 5 minutes until the onion is translucent then stir in the spinach. Season with salt and pepper to taste.
6. Cook for 1 to 2 minutes more until the spinach is wilted then spoon the mixture over the mushroom caps to serve.

Servings: 4

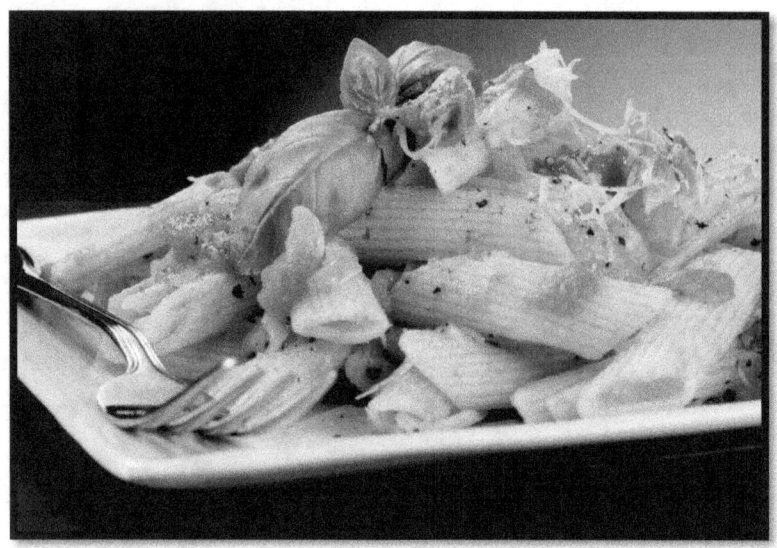

Ingredients:

10 ounces whole wheat pasta

1 tablespoon olive oil

2 cloves garlic, minced

1 small yellow onion, chopped

3 cups fresh diced tomatoes

¼ cup fresh chopped basil

1 teaspoon dried oregano

Salt and pepper to taste

Instructions:

1. Bring a large pot of salted water to boil and add the pasta.
2. Cook the pasta until al dente, about 9 to 11 minutes, then drain and set aside to keep warm.
3. Meanwhile, heat the oil in a medium saucepan over medium heat.
4. Add the onion and garlic then cook for 5 minutes until the onion is translucent – season with salt and pepper to taste.
5. Stir in the tomatoes and bring to a boil then reduce heat and simmer for 10 minutes.
6. Transfer the sauce to a food processor and add the basil and oregano.
7. Blend the mixture until smooth then serve over the cooked pasta.

Grilled Veggie and Tofu Kebabs

Servings: 6

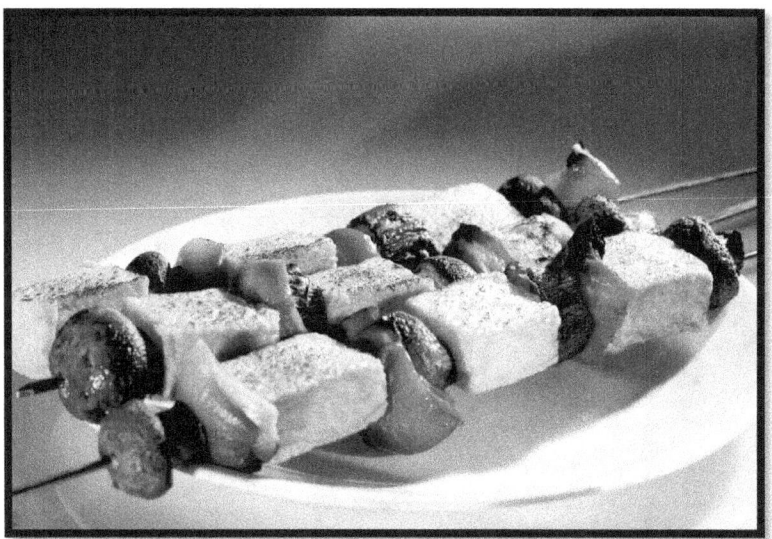

Ingredients:

1 teaspoon minced garlic

¼ cup fresh chopped chives

2 tablespoons olive oil

1 ½ tablespoons fresh lemon juice

2 teaspoons apple cider vinegar

2 tablespoons water

½ small avocado, pitted and chopped

Salt and pepper to taste

1 (14 ounce) package extra-firm tofu, cut into 1-inch cubes

1 red bell pepper, cored and cut into 1-inch chunks

1 green bell pepper, cored and cut into 1-inch chunks

1 large red onion, cut into 1-inch chunks

1 cup button mushrooms, cleaned

Wooden skewers, soaked overnight

Olive oil, as needed

Instructions:

1. Combine the garlic, chives, olive oil, lemon juice, apple cider vinegar and water in a small mixing bowl.

2. Place the avocado in a food processor and blend smooth. Season with salt and pepper to taste.
3. Add the garlic mixture and blend until smooth and creamy – add water, if needed, to thin.
4. Preheat the grill to medium-low heat and brush the grates with olive oil.
5. Slide the vegetables and tofu cubes onto the skewers and brush with oil.
6. Set the kebabs on the grill and cook for 12 to 15 minutes, turning every 5 minutes, until the kebabs are lightly charred.
7. Transfer the kebabs to a serving platter and drizzle with dressing to serve.

Servings: 4

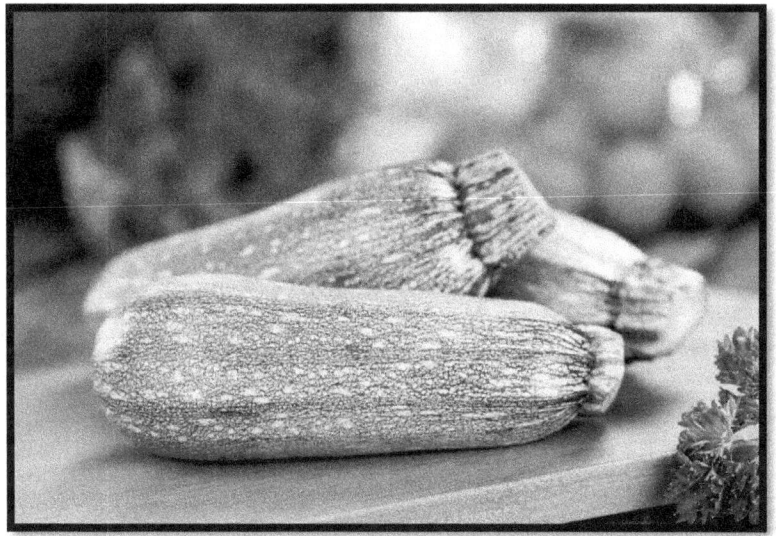

Ingredients:

2 medium zucchini

1 tablespoon fresh lemon juice

1 tablespoon coconut oil

½ small yellow onion, diced

1 tablespoon fresh minced garlic

2 tablespoons fresh chopped parsley

Instructions:

1. Peel the zucchini into ribbon-like threads using a vegetable peeler or spiralizer.
2. Toss the zucchini with lemon juice and set aside.
3. Heat the oil in a medium skillet over medium heat.
4. Add the onion and garlic and cook for 4 to 5 minutes, stirring often.
5. Toss in the zucchini noodles and cook for 2 to 3 minutes until just heated through.
6. Garnish with fresh chopped parsley to serve.

Servings: 4

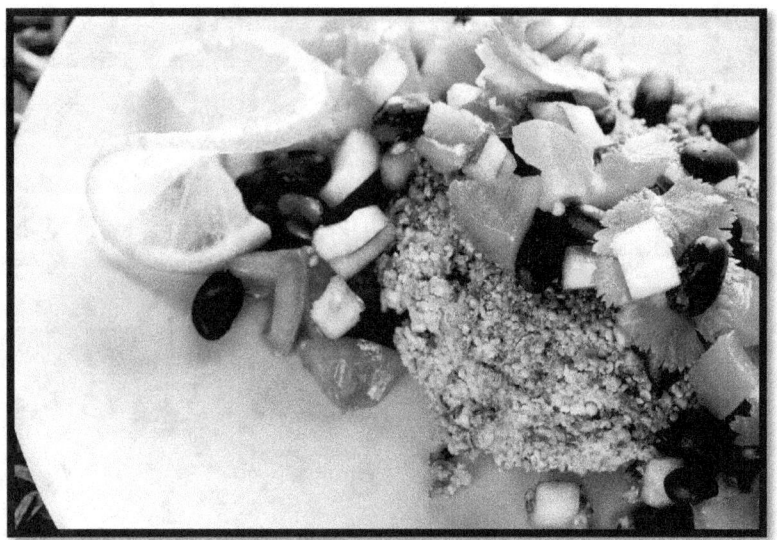

Ingredients:

2 tablespoons ground flaxseed
3 tablespoons warm water
2 (15.5 ounce) cans black beans
¾ cup ground almond meal
½ small white onion, diced
Salt and pepper to taste

Instructions:

1. Whisk together the ground flaxseed and warm water in a small bowl then let rest for 5 to 10 minutes.
2. Drain the black beans and place them in a bowl then mash them using a fork or the back of a wooden spoon.
3. Stir in the almond meal, onion, flax egg, salt and pepper then stir well.
4. Let the mixture sit for 5 minutes then shape by hand into four even-sized patties.
5. Heat a large skillet over medium heat and grease with cooking spray.
6. Add the patties and cook for 5 minutes on each side until cooked through and browned on the outside.
7. Serve on whole-wheat sandwich buns with your favorite burger toppings.

Conclusion

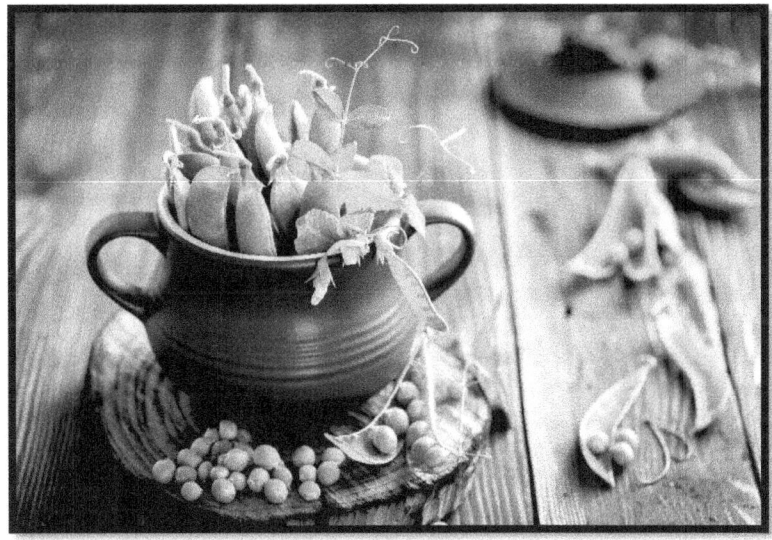

After reading this book you should have a basic understanding of what the Daniel Fast Diet is and how to follow it. You should also have an understanding of the benefits the Daniel Fast Diet may have in store for you. In following this diet you will engage in healthy eating principles which will improve your overall nutrient and it may also spark healthy weight loss. If you choose to incorporate the spiritual component of the diet, you may also receive a deeper level of spirituality and a closer communion with God. If you think that the Daniel Fast Diet is truly the right choice for you, head to the grocery store and get started with one of the easy 15-minute recipes provided in this book!

www.ingramcontent.com/pod-product-compliance
Lightning Source LLC
Chambersburg PA
CBHW080740290526

45790CB00008B/3266